PELVIS WORKOUT MANUAL

ULTIMATE STEP BY STEP GUIDE ON PELVIC WORKOUT

DR. GLENN HAGARD

Table of Contents

CHAPTER ONE

Workouts for the Pelvis

Kegel exercises are what they sound like.

This type of exercise, called a kegel, helps to strengthen the muscles in your pelvic floor. Your reproductive organs are housed in the region between your hips, which is called your pelvis.

At the bottom of your pelvis, you have a hammock-like structure of muscles and tissues known as the "pelvic floor." The sling secures your internal organs. Incontinence or inability to control one's bowels or bladder can be the result of a weak pelvic floor.

You can practice Kegel exercises in the privacy of your own home, or while waiting in line at the bank, as long as you understand them.

What's the point of doing Kegel exercises?

Kegel exercises are beneficial to both sexes.

Pregnancy, childbirth, aging, and weight gain are just a few of the things that can weaken a woman's pelvic floor.

Supporting the womb, bladder, and bowels is the pelvic floor muscle group. It is possible for these pelvic organs to fall into the vagina of a woman who has weak muscles. Urinary incontinence is a possible side effect, in addition to the discomfort.

As we get older, the muscles in our pelvic floor can weaken, too.

For men with prostate surgery, this can lead to incontinence of both urine and stool.

Identifying the muscles of the pelvic floor in women

Finding the right set of muscles for Kegel exercises can be difficult when you first begin. Place a finger inside your vagina and tighten the muscles around the finger to find them.

You can also try to stop your urine mid-flow in order to find the muscles. Your pelvic floor muscles are the ones you use to perform this action. Become familiar with the sensations that arise as a result of contracting and relaxing your muscles.

However, this method should only be used for educational purposes. You should avoid starting and stopping your urine frequently, or doing Kegel exercises frequently, when your bladder is full. A urinary tract infection can increase your risk of incomplete bladder emptying (UTI).

If you're still unsure about which muscles to target, make an appointment with your gynecologist. Using an object called a vaginal cone may be recommended by them. The pelvic floor muscles are used to keep a vaginal cone in place after it is inserted into the vagina.

Pelvic floor muscle identification and isolation can be facilitated through biofeedback training. A small probe is inserted into your vagina or adhesive electrodes are applied to the outside of your vagina or anus during this procedure. A Kegel will be required of you. The length of time you were able to hold the contraction will be displayed on the monitor.

Men's pelvic floor muscles: what to look for

Even in men, it's not always easy to identify the correct group of pelvic floor muscles. Inserting a finger into the rectum and trying to squeeze it, without tightening the muscles of the abdomen, buttocks or legs, is one way to find them for men.

Tensing the muscles that prevent you from passing gas can also be beneficial.

Use a stop-and-go method if you're still having issues. This is a reliable method for finding the pelvic floor muscles in men, but it should not be used on a regular basis.

Males can benefit from biofeedback as well. It's possible that you may need to see your doctor if you can't find them on your own.

Kegel training's objectives and benefits

Before beginning Kegel exercises, make sure your bladder is completely empty. Before beginning your exercises, find a quiet, private spot to sit or lie down. You'll be able to perform them anywhere once you've practiced them enough.

CHAPTER TWO

To begin Kegel exercises, tense the muscles in your pelvic floor for three counts, then relax them for the same number of counted-out periods of time. Don't stop until you've completed a full set of 10. Spend the next few days working on your muscle tension until you can hold it for a count of ten. Every day, you should aim to complete three sets of ten repetitions.

If you don't see results right away, don't get discouraged. According to the Mayo Clinic, the effects of Kegel exercises on urinary incontinence can take up to a few months.

Each person experiences them in a unique way. Muscle control and urinary continence are two areas in which some people have shown significant improvement. Kegels, on the other hand, may keep your condition from worsening.

Cautions

After a Kegel exercise session, if you feel pain in your abdomen or back, this indicates that you're not doing them correctly. Be sure to keep the muscles of your back and sides as loose as possible, even as you tighten your pelvic floor muscles.

Don't overdo it with the Kegels, either. If you overwork your muscles, they will become fatigued and unable to carry out their essential tasks.

There are many benefits to performing kegel exercises to strengthen the muscles in the pelvis, bladder, and bowel. Urinary and bowel control issues can affect both men and women. The following may be a problem for you:

— As you grow older

• If you put on weight,

After the birth of a child

Following surgery on the uterus (women)

- After a prostatic procedure (men)

Neurological and psychiatric conditions can cause urinary and bowel incontinence.

Any time you're sitting or lying down is a good time to do kegel exercises. Work, rest, and entertainment all qualify as acceptable times to perform these tasks.

How to Identify the Right Muscles for Your Goal

Pretend to have to urinate and hold it for as long as you can during a Kegel exercise. You tense and relax the muscles that control the flow of urine in order to relieve yourself. Finding the correct muscles to tighten is critical.

Try starting to go and then stopping the next time you have to urinate. Tighten and raise the muscles in your vagina, bladder, or anus (for females). These are the muscles of the pelvic floor. You've done the exercise correctly if you can feel your muscles tightening. Your thighs, buttocks, and abdomen should all remain supple and unstrained.

When in doubt, here are some additional tips to ensure you're focusing on the correct muscle groups:

Assume that you're trying to avoid passing gas at all costs.

In the case of females, place a fingertip inside the vaginal opening. As if you were trying to hold in your pee, contract your muscles and then relax them.

Muscles that move up and down and tighten should be felt.

In the case of males, place a finger in the rectum. Let go of the muscles as if you were squeezing your bladder. You should be able to feel the muscles contract and move in and out.

Exercises for the Kegel

Do Kegel exercises three times a day once you have a sense of how the movement should feel:

Sit or lie down after making sure your bladder is empty.

• Engage your pelvic floor muscles by contracting them. Hold your breath for 3 to 5 seconds, then release.

Breathe deeply and focus on your breathing for 3 to 5 seconds.

At least three times per day should be done (morning, afternoon, and night).

While performing these exercises, be sure to take deep

breaths and relax your entire body. Do not tighten the muscles in your stomach, thighs, buttocks, or chest while doing this.........

You should feel better and experience fewer symptoms after 4 to 6 weeks. Do the exercises as directed, but do not up the ante in terms of repetitions. Struggling to urinate or move your bowels is a sign that you've gone too far.

Here are a few warnings:

Do not practice Kegel exercises while you are urinating more than twice a month after learning how to do them. Performing the exercises while urinating can weaken your pelvic floor muscles or damage your bladder and kidneys over time..

A woman's vaginal muscles may tighten too much if she performs Kegel exercises incorrectly or with a lot of force. Sexual intercourse can be painful as a result of this.

If you stop doing these exercises, your incontinence will return. You may have to keep doing them for the rest of your life if you start now.

Incontinence can take months to go away if you start doing these exercises.

To whom should you go for help?

If you have any doubts about whether or not you are performing Kegel exercises correctly, speak with your doctor. You can have your provider check to see if you're doing them right. Referrals for pelvic floor exercises may be made by your doctor.

CHAPTER THREE

Step-by-step instructions on how to perform kegels.

You won't look any better doing Kegel exercises, but you will strengthen the muscles that support your bladder, which is just as important. In the fight against incontinence, a well-trained pelvic floor muscles can make all the difference.

Despite the fact that Kegel exercises are easy to perform,

finding the right muscles to target is not. Kegels work the muscles in the abdomen, buttocks, and inner thighs of about one-third of people who perform them. The exercises have no effect on them.

Locate the muscles in your pelvis.

Finding the right muscles to work out on can be accomplished through the use of a variety of methods.

Women:

Try to avoid passing gas as if you were trying to avoid it.

Tighten your vagina around a tampon as if it were a tampon.

Men:

Try to avoid passing gas as if you were trying to avoid it.

During the process of urination, try to stop the flow of your own urine.

Your pelvic muscles will contract more in the back than the front if you've identified and activated the right ones.

Make use of the contractions.

Your position is up to you. Lie on your back for a few minutes to get a feel for the contractions of the pelvic floor. Once you've got the hang of it, switch between standing and sitting practice.

Relax and contract

For 3 to 5 seconds, contract your pelvic floor muscles.

- Take a few deep breaths.

Ten times through the cycle of contracting and relaxing.

Keep the rest of your muscles loose. Keep your abdominal, leg, and buttock muscles relaxed, and don't raise your pelvis during the exercise. When you feel a movement in your abdomen, gently place your hand on it.

Expend your vacation period. Increase the duration of the contractions and relaxations over time. Work your way up to ten-second contractions and relaxations, one at a time.

The sky's the limit. Every day, do at least 30 to 40 Kegel exercises to keep your pelvic floor strong and healthy. Instead of doing everything at once, spread them out over the course of the day. It's easy to sneak in a few of these stealth exercises while waiting at a stoplight, riding an elevator, or standing in a supermarket line.

Diversify. Short contractions and releases (sometimes referred to as "quick flicks") should be practiced alongside longer ones.

Performing Kegel exercises in the event of a medical emergency

For people who suffer from stress incontinence, one or more Kegel exercises may be all that is needed to prevent any leakage when the "trigger" occurs. Doing Kegels may help you get to the bathroom if you're afraid you won't be able to get there in time.

Things to Keep an Eye Out For

Between Kegels, the pelvic floor muscles need to be relaxed, and this is just as important as the squeezing motions.

There are many ways to look at this. For example, when you

practice Kegels, you're strengthening your muscles so that you can, for example, close your genitals on command. Your muscles will be unable to tighten further in times of need if you are constantly clamping down. In a similar way, if you always keep your hand in a fist, it becomes difficult to grab onto something when the time comes.

When doing Kegels, avoid squeezing or tightening any of the adjacent muscles, such as those in your stomach, buttocks, or lower legs. The pelvic muscles can be hampered if you do this. It's also possible that tightening the muscles around the pelvic floor, rather than the actual pelvic floor muscles, will put pressure on your bladder.

THE END

www.ingramcontent.com/pod-product-compliance
Lightning Source LLC
LaVergne TN
LVHW010124170826
845678LV00012B/2583

* 9 7 9 8 8 4 5 8 4 5 4 8 1 *